"SENIOR SEASON"

"Aging with Grace"

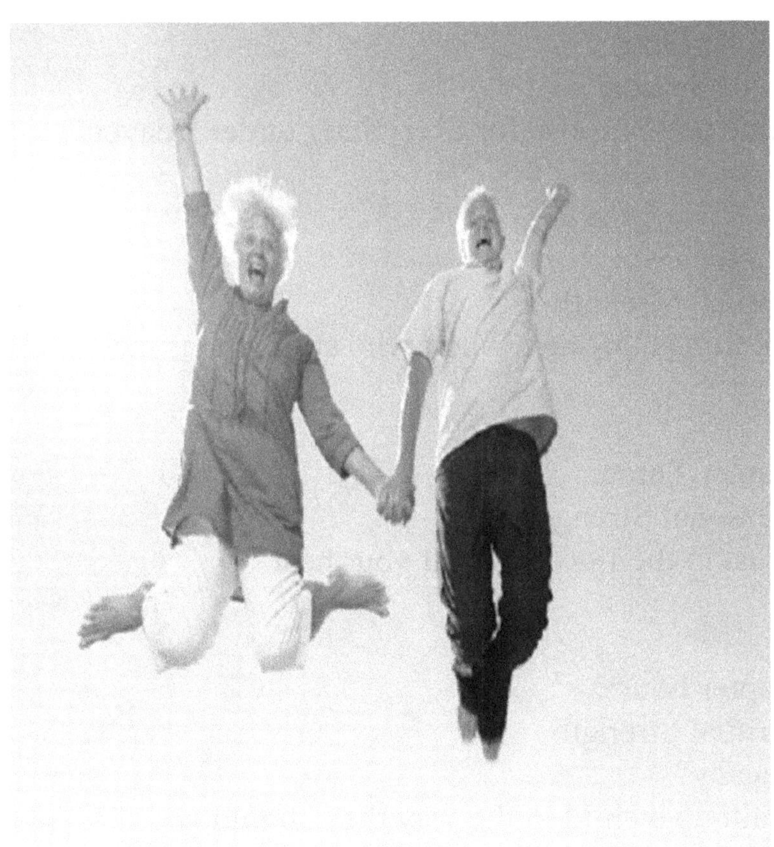

TABLE OF CONTENTS:

Introduction

Chapter One:
Senior Season
"Time and purpose for everything under Heaven."

Chapter Two:
Physical Strength
"All things through Christ who strengthens me"

Chapter Three:
Emotional Strength
"Trust in the Lord with all your heart"

Chapter Four:
Spiritual Strength
"Legacy"
"Train up a child in the way they should go"

Introduction

Many of my previous books have been about different seasons of life I have been going through. Actually they were seasons that the Lord Jesus has been taking me through and moving me forward. This book is no different talking, battling, defeating, and propelling through this senior season. This season of coming of old age, of retirement, of future, of completing the purpose that God has placed me on this earth.

I hesitate in referring to this of old age. I really want it to be a season of promise, of health, of vitality, of purpose, and of legacy. Even with the pain that I seem to be going through, the natural deterioration of the body, the gray hair, muscle loss, and all the other health concerns that seem to keep cropping up as you grow older. With all the above said, I do not want to confess the issues of aging or be defined by those physical and emotional concerns that seem to be all so natural. In the natural our tendency may to be focusing how we are closer to death and the end of our life, but I want my focus to be on life, not death. Our tendency may to be that we are older and more frail, but I want to focus on being strong, not weak. We may think that we are at the end of our life, but I would rather believe we are at the beginning of a new joyous and exciting season. Our final season of life has many possibilities and promise if we approach life in a different manner, attitude, and lifestyle. We have the opportunity to go out with a bang.

If we look into scripture and the Word of God, even the first book of Genesis talks about Adam who lived 930 years, Noah lived to 950 years, Abraham lived to 175 years, and Moses to 120 years. God created man to never die, but sin crept in and brought forth death. (James 1:14) God also said in Genesis 6:3-5 "My Spirit will not strive with man for he is flesh and that the wickedness of man was great in the earth and every imagination of the thoughts of their heart were evil continually, so his days shall be 120 years." Even though initially man was made to never die, sin and evil crept in and God put a limit on our flesh and bodies to 120 years. His word is true even though right now there isn't many who even live to 120, but that is the limit and time set by God. That time did come to pass for you can see above from the time to Noah of 950 years to Moses, time decreased to 120. That took may years to be fulfilled, but once spoken, our time in this life did decrease.

Well, I am currently 60, so with that in mind I may have 20 days to 20 years left. No man knows the time of his passing or the fulfillment of his life. Tomorrow is promised to no one and we have to be focused on today with the future in preparation. Believing I have twenty years, there is much I can do and much I still can accomplish, and there is much for you to do and accomplish also. Going through the Bible, You will see that God used older mature men most of the time to fulfill his purpose on the earth. Not true always, but many times. I want to be like Caleb who was with Joshua entering the promised land. (Joshua 14) Caleb's statement to Joshua was; "The Lord has kept me alive this fourscore and five years, and I am as strong as I was at forty five, Give me this mountain for my inheritance." Four score and five years equates to eighty years old. Caleb's confession was he was strong at this age and he climbed a Mountain. Caleb felt as strong at 85 as he did at 45.

It is funny how God speaks to us. He speaks in his word for sure, he speaks through others in your life including children, He speaks through your spirit and conscience, and he speaks to me often in songs. I hear many different songs when I wake that encourage me and also guide and direct me. We think everything has to be super spiritual, but God spoke to me before this book with a George Jones' Classic:

"I don't need your rocking chair,
Your Geritol or your Medicare.
I still got Neon in my veins,
This gray hair don't mean a thing.
I do my rocking on a stage,
Can't put this possum in a cage,
My bodies old but it ain't impaired,
I Don't Need your Rocking Chair!"

That is the confession I want to have in these coming years; to scale and conquer mountains just as Caleb did.

We can all have that confession, the Lord will give us that strength if we just confess, believe, and press forward. Moving forward should be our focus not being stagnant. We need to be physically fit, emotionally strong, and spiritually ready to take those mountains. That is what this book is all about. The Bible has much information and encouragement for us to accomplish all we desire to accomplish for him. We have much wisdom to give our children and grandchildren. We have strength to serve our Church and our Community. We were made to live and were made to give life. We have much to give and many who are retired have much time to do so. We are going to go further in this book on the wisdom God has revealed to me and also steps we can take to achieve our lifelong purpose and legacy.

Chapter One
Senior Season
"Time and purpose for everything under Heaven"

This is almost an introduction after the intro. I haven't to this point of my writing really finalized the title of this book. I am looking at senior season at this time but it may change as I am writing. In fact, I have written other chapters before I have even written this one. The scripture above came to my heart and spirit while in this writing. This scripture is found in Ecclesiastes 3:1; "To everything there is a season and a time to every purpose under Heaven." This was even a song in the sixties written that many who read this book will remember; "Turn, Turn, Turn". Statistically, those of us in our senior season is increasing in number. There are almost 50 million of those 65 or older. In Canada, we number 1 of every six persons. We are not only surviving and living longer, we are thriving!

The Book of Ecclesiastes goes on to say there is a time to be born and a time to die, a time to weep and a time to mourn, a time to gather and a time to cast away, a time to get and a time to lose, and a time to weep and mourn and a time to laugh and dance among others. A season as defined in the dictionary naturally talks about spring, summer, winter, and fall. It also talks about time for certain activities, time valid for certain time, to become adapted, and to grow to fit to use. In the Bible season refers to all the above but also an appointed time, an opportunity, place of meeting and a chronological step.

I stand in awe in all those definitions because if you think about each of your life steps and seasons all of then are involved. Through life we have went through many different seasons from our youth, to teens, to middle aged, to married with kids, from childhood to adult. Each and every season we had gone through had a purpose and place in our lives, a meaning to how we came to who we are. Each individual season was a preparation for the next season. Each season brought teaching and learning and growth. Each season was like a stepping stone to the next level and season.

We may feel that our growth and learning are done in our senior season. We may feel that we have accomplished most of what we may have wanted to in life, or we may feel that we didn't accomplish anything we set out to do. In this season of life I believe that all of that is true. In this season of life we still have much to learn and much to grow and much to give. If you look at the word senior, at this age you may be thinking senior citizen which in most terms means old or aged. But I like to look at the word as meaning mature, superior in stature, or the higher class like a senior in high school; one who has graduated and ready to go to the next level and conquer the world. If you look at those definitions of senior, you will begin to believe that there is much more to come and much more to do.

The phrase "Bucket List" has become really popular. A list of everything you would like to do or places you would like to go before your passing. A lot of that list may be made up of possible daredevil feats such as sky diving, zip lining, or a number of other things. I have been blessed to drive fast in cars, snowmobiles, and motorcycles; living life on the edge and sometimes foolishly. I have water skied and skied on snow. There are a few things I would like to do even at this age to include zip lining or maybe riding in a air balloon. My wife is not as adventurous but she would like to travel more as I would also. She would like to go to a working ranch and ride horses. I would like to travel to Israel among others. Everyone of us has a bucket list and everyone of us has a different item on that list. That list is encouraged in us to live and to have life in our senior season. The Lord created the seasons! The Lord created morning and night, days, weeks, months and years. He created the sun and the moon which direct the four seasons of summer, winter, fall, and spring. (Genesis1) Genesis 1 is the first book of the Bible and the first things God did is created all the above. He created and orchestrated each and every season in our life, and we are to give Him Glory in living out each and every season to the best we can, and that included this senior season. This season is not the end, but a new beginning for new things.

It is amazing when you look above at the different seasons we can find ourselves in. Summer, Winter, Fall, and Spring, but there is also days, weeks, months, and years; Seasons within a season. You could have a separate season within a season. One thing for certain is each and every season brings change. I have to admit that I struggle with change sometimes. My wife even jokes I am in a box occasionally. I like my chair in the same place. Moving and rearranging the Living Room is bad for me. I do need to learn to embrace change sometimes, because a lot of good things can happen when we are taken out of our comfort zones, on the other side of the coin sometimes things get rougher also.

We just moved into a new home and that was a great change. We also got a new car and I am way happier with that change. A new job and new friends are also great changes at times. While I am writing this, one of our son's and grandchildren are moving fifty miles away. I am pretty depressed over that change and it will be hard to adapt to this. For ten years we were within miles and seeing and being involved with their lives was easy. We are blessed that we live as close as fifty miles with three of our sons and grandchildren, but right now fifty miles seems like 500.

We will adapt and make different plans to see each other, but it goes back to maybe some of the reason I don't like change. I know everything will work out, it always has, but we realize and know that change can be a great thing and also a hard thing. Change whether we want to admit it happens continuously and constantly no matter what season we are in or entering into. One way to adapt to change is to not just react to change, but to be the change. We can always choose to make a change for the better thus creating change and not reacting to change. Change is defined as an alteration or alternative to what is already going on. It is a shift that happens, not always a complete 180. Also, just because we experience change doesn't mean it affects every aspect of our life, usually just a portion, and that I and also you can deal with.

A good example about being a change goes with my issue above. Whether your loved ones are 50 or 500 miles away, we can still stay in contact, we can still let them know that we are thinking about them. It is not hard to call or sent a text or message. My wife is good about calling and it gets returned often. She is constantly and continually on phone with our kids. I am not good on phones, something I got from my own father. When I called home, he said; "Hi, how are you doing, need anything, here is your mother." But, obviously I can write and my staying in contact is in that manner. My feelings and emotions are better displayed in this manner of written communication rather than by spoken words.

Chapter Two:
Physical Strength
"All things through Christ who strengthens me"

If we have any limitations when we are older, our physical strength would be the category. We are not as strong as we were when we were twenty to thirty years old. Our mind still thinks like a twenty to thirty year old (more on this in the emotional part of this book), but our bodies really are not the same. Our metabolism is not as fast, our muscle tone is not the same, and our bodies are not as strong. Not only is our muscle tone not the same, but our skin starts to wrinkle, and our head and hair is turning gray. Again, at twenty to thirty years old, I believe you are at your prime physically; in youth, looks, and outer beauty. Even though I want to be strong and full of vigor, our bodies are failing little by little. It is the natural aging process that we try to fight but the reality is we are not as strong as we used to be. Still gray hair is known in the Bible as one who has experience and wisdom. Truthfully, age gives us experience, but God gives wisdom. (We will address this in Spiritual Strength Chapter) We have been through a few things and have earned every one of our gray hairs, lol.

With that said, we still need to be the best we can be at the stage of life we find ourselves in. I am going to reference my condition many times but I feel that most of us in this senior stage are going through these concerns and situations. Keep in mind that I am not a health, fitness, or nutrition expert; just does what works for me. In my case, I would probably be in better health if I took care of myself better when I was younger. I joke that if I knew I was going to live this long, I would have taken better care of myself when I was younger. When we are younger we think we do not have limitations and we push ourselves even past the limits we may have had then. I burned the candle at both ends, ate and drank whatever I wanted, and did whatever I wanted. Even though I was very active, I didn't do focused exercise much. Many of the injuries I had when I was younger, I feel the effects even now as I am older.

For me, I feel I take way to much medication. I am prescribed medications for Blood Pressure, Cholesterol, and pain and muscle relaxing medications for my arthritis. For me at this stage if life, the medication gets me by day to day. I am always believing for better health and healing, but until then take what is needed to get me to the next day. My wife has diabetes and we still believe and hope for her healing but she does what she needs to in watching her diet and taking her insulin getting by day to day. We need to take things day to day and maybe that is the better way to look at life even as seniors, live for today but plan for tomorrow. The Bible tells us which is good medicine; "Take no thought for tomorrow for tomorrow will take care of itself, sufficient is the task and duties for today." (Matthew 6:34) Thinking about tomorrow many times brings worries, but focusing on today brings purpose. It is not bad to be concerned, but we have to be careful not to be consumed. I know personally when I think about it and think about the past, everything worked out and was taken care of. That is where we need to be now. Again, statistically it is known that actually most seniors have less stress. They differentiate needs from wants more clearly and more clear and focused goals. Although always important to some extent, we care less about what someone thinks of us.

As I am older, I know that proper exercise, nutrition and eating habits, and plenty of sleep are needed and beneficial for me to have the vim and vigor I need at this age to do all the tasks I need to accomplish in a given day, week, or month. There are still limitations with my exercise, but I try to exercise two to three times a week. For me at this stage, I do rope training. I have arthritis in my joints and this exercise doesn't harm my joints but does strengthen my muscles. I try to walk daily which is easy in the summertime but harder in this Northern Michigan climate. My wife is not one for daily exercise, but she is active every day. It is all I can do sometimes to keep up with her. She was raised a farm girl and that work ethic keeps her moving everyday whether taking care of me or taking care of kids and grand-kids. As important as exercise is, I truly believe proper nutrition is more important. For me, I love my meat especially grilling. In fact most of my friends and family would admit that I just love to eat. It is one of the Lord's bounties that I enjoy very much, but even my father said everything is good unless it is overdone. We all have to watch our intake of food, eating more vegetables and fruits. Like I said, I am not a nutritionist but every weight loss program and nutritionist all agree more fruits and vegetables. They also say lean meat eating more chicken than beef. For me again, if I start to gain weight it is because of starches; breads and potatoes. If I limit those, My weight will stay stable. Luckily, my wife has to watch starches and sugars, so our meal plan has that in mind for both of us.

The big danger I believe and it is constantly coming out in articles is sugars. Sugars which are suppose to give you energy, drain you and actually too much makes me feel sick. Our bodies created by God have the ability to tell us if we are not living right and eating right. Here it is after the Holidays and my body is screaming at me to change my lifestyle and eating habits. Food has the ability to make us feel great or to make us very unhealthy if not monitored properly. Right now after the holidays, my choice is to quit eating so much sugar in the form of desserts and cookies and cakes. Even that one change will make a significant difference. That is awesome that no matter your age, just making one lifestyle change can make a miraculous change on how we feel. The Bible calls this fasting! Actually true fasting is denying yourself to get closer to God, denying your fleshly appetites to increase your spiritual awareness. Truthfully, biblical fasting could be one meal or not eating for a day or not eating for up to forty days. Surprisingly I am also writing this at the time of lent. Many are familiar with lent especially if raised Catholic which I was. I now consider myself Conservative Christian seeking the Kingdom of God and His Son. But still the principal of fasting is known and observed in all walks of life. Fasting could also include not watching the news, television, or participating in social media; whatever draws you closer to God and away from the troubles of the world. Nutritionists still agree, abstaining from food for even one day will cleanse your system so the principals God gives us works. If we focus on healthy eating we bring us health that is needed especially in our age bracket.

My wife and my son drink water like there is no tomorrow. I try to do this as it is recommended to drink a gallon of water a day. I don't keep track of the amount or measure of water I drink but try to drink a glass an hour. There is nothing that will flush your system like water. There is nothing more refreshing to you than cool clear water. Water is necessary for life, for all life whether plant or animal. Natural water brings our bodies life, flushes out toxins and enhances our systems. Jesus talking to the woman at the well said; "Whoever drinks of this natural water will thirst again, but whoever drinks of the water I give shall never thirst; but the water

I give them shall be a well of water springing up to eternal life." (John 4) Jesus also repeated in John 7:38; "He that believes in me, out of his belly shall flow rivers of living water." Water is necessary and crucial in natural but is just as important in the Spiritual. Water gives life in natural but also gives life in the Spirit. The Holy Spirit is symbolized not only as a dove, but also as living water, not water itself as we know it, but a refreshing of our spirit.

What we need to all focus on is not being stagnant and sitting through this stage of life. Rest and relaxation is good but overdone, I actually feel worse not doing something. I know a person who has been setting in a lounge chair for most of her later years and all she mentions is how much pain she is in. In our later years we have earned this extra rest and relaxation, and there are even days I take a short nap to better myself. I enjoy them and they give me that extra I need some days. I am not fully retired at this age and still work part time in a warehouse. I find in doing that I feel better, I may not feel I can do a forty to fifty hour workweek, but part time work keeps us active. It is not only beneficial physically but also mentally. I can see me working part time probably till the day I die. It still gives me plenty of time to do what I want or volunteer, or take time writing books. Again, what works for me may not be the answer for every one out there, but the point I am trying to make is to keep as active as you can to stay as active as we need to be. Maybe for some, it is biking, jogging, or swimming, but whatever works like Nike says, Just do it!

"Do you not know that your body is the temple of the Holy Ghost which is in you, which you have of God and you are not your own." (I Corinthians 6:19) The Bible says our bodies are a temple! A temple first because when we accept Jesus into our heart as savior, the Holy Spirit of God comes to live inside each and every one of us. That is a awesome relationship spiritually, but our bodies are a temple naturally also. That means to take care of your body to the best of your ability. It is one of God's greatest creation. You were fearfully and wonderfully made in his image. One of the things the Lord reminds me to do is pamper myself. That means not only eating right and exercising, but to also take care of the little things, even as much as getting a haircut rejuvenates us. Things as simple as trimming nails, hand lotions, and bathing. Relaxing in a hot tub, resting, and getting physically and spiritually renewed. We will talk more about this in our chapter on Spiritual Strength. Taking time for yourself is not selfish. You can only help others when you are the best you can be and that means at times to pamper ourselves at times. In this season by taking proper care of ourselves we are not only adding years to our life, but life to our years.

"I can do all things through Christ who strengthens me." (Philippians 4:13) That is a good confession, instruction, and also a good inspiration. There are many times we all need supernatural strength. Christ gives us the extra strength we need many times; in infirmities (sickness), in distress (dark days), persecution (trouble), and in necessities (when ever necessary). (II Corinthians 12:10) We will find ourselves in those trials whether young or old and we need to admit to ourselves that there are many times and many things we cannot do on our own, but also need to believe that there is always help in any time of need. The Lord has been faithful through out my entire life to help in my every need. He is no respecter of persons, so if he did it for me, he will do it for you. "Blessed be the Lord my strength who trains my hands for war." (Psalm 144:1) This was the confession of King David who was one of God's great warriors. David knew where his strength came from when he went to war or battle. You may not be in a war, but many days we are in a battle and we can rely on the strength of our God.

One day we are all going to die whether from sickness, age, or accident. Death comes to young and old, rich and poor, and plays no favorites. I do not know why I have lived as long as I have and I question why many babies and children and young have gone before me. I have lived foolishly at times and still am alive. The Lord purposes for each of us seventy years and possibly eighty with his strength. (Psalm 91:10) We are people who the Lord has given us free will and that in the midst of a sin has brought forth death. It is not the Lord's will babies die in abortion, or children to die of disease, or even people to die because of a drunk driver, but it happens. There are many things we do not and cannot understand this side of Heaven. I know all of our time is limited and we are to make the best of it we can while we are given each and every day. Each day is a gift not a given right. The Bible says even seventy years is a like a vapor or puff of smoke. Life on this earth goes by fast. It seems like yesterday I just got married even though I have been married thirty years. It seems I was just enjoying the birth of my sons even though they are now young men who are married and have children of their own. Death in this life is coming but eternal life is also what we have to look forward to through Jesus. (John 3:16 / 17:3)

Chapter Three:
Emotional Strength
"Trust in the Lord with all your heart"

Emotional strength is defined as the mind, the will, and emotions. It is said you are only as young as you feel. That has to do with the mind primarily in our perceptions and our attitude. Our feelings have to do with our emotions but also our heart. That twelve inch space between our heart and mind, getting both our feelings and our thoughts together can be difficult sometimes. Although we are senior citizens we still have the heart of a child and the mind of a twenty year old. We have everything around us telling us we are old, but everything inside us saying we still feel young. That is one of the battles going on with our heart, mind and bodies. That is the reason for emotional strength in this senior season and the reason for this chapter in this book.

There are a lot of things going on in our minds right now. I have many concerns and thoughts during this time and season. Truthfully, no matter what season of life I found myself in I had thoughts and concerns; whether they were when I first got married, having our first child, buying our first home, or many other issues. Another truth is thoughts that turn into concerns turn into worries. It is fine to meditate, resolve and address issues and thoughts, but when they turn to worries, we have thought too far. We move into stinking thinking.

We get consumed on what may happen to what is happening. I have said it before and will say it again, when I look back on my life; everything worked out, maybe not always how I thought or planned but still most came out fine. I Peter 5:7 says; "Cast all our cares (concerns) on the Lord for he cares for you." If we learn to just trust in the Lord and go about our daily activities he directs our path. He is a lamp to our feet and a light to our path. He illuminates our path and gives us direction step by step.

There are many things I am personally concerned with and think about a lot during this season. Maybe you find yourselves in the same place or maybe you have totally others that are different. One of the major concerns I have at this stage of life is finances which I am sure there are many out there with the same issues. My wife and I live on a budget and a limited income, but our needs are met everyday. We have food, clothing, and a new home. I joke that at sixty I have a new mortgage, but I am happy with our new house. In our life we went from having a farm to an apartment to a modular home to a house. It is a book in itself if I told you the story on how God orchestrated this blessing. We went through many houses, but as it is important to have a place to lay your head, houses will crumble and be in need of continuous repair, but a home is forever. A house is just a empty building, but a home brings love, children, family, and life. A house or residence is temporary, but a home is forever. The value of a house is in its structure, but the value of a home is what is found inside.

Financially when I was younger I thought I had this all figured out. I had retirement concern back when I was thirty and started a 401K plan which many others have probably done also. I actually started and was building a good retirement until 2008 when stocks, housing, banking, and jobs collapsed. For many years I was making a great living over sixty thousand a year, of course much of that to finance our family and lifestyle and house we were living in. It is amazing that here in the United States no matter how much we make we increase our style of living to match our income instead of saving for a rainy day and a future income. With the 401K I thought I had the future planned though. Anyways, along comes 2008 where I lost my job. In the process we also lost the farm we had which was hard on my wife since this was kind of her heritage. See, we can plan and think we have everything figured out, but in just one day everything could change and go south. There are no guarantees in this world like they say except death and taxes. To some extent there is truth to that. No matter how hard we work and or plan sometimes things will fail. One day things went from stable to unstable but many times in life it also goes the other way, from bad to great. It really wasn't a surprise when all this started happening because God told me months before in preparation this was going to happen. That is one of the greatest things about having a relationship with the Lord is that he prepares us for what is to come. He also tries to show us ways to be better prepared like saving more but I have to admit I didn't listen good enough to that one. I wasn't overly concerned because I knew God had a plan and it always was a better plan.

It was a very difficult time nonetheless for I was unemployed for four years. There were many miracles of provision and transition during this time. When 2008 hit, we had a 150,000 dollar mortgage and ashamed to say, heavy credit card debt. With all we went through in the midst of lack we lost our home and farm, but also was able to come out of this seven year transition debt free. It was a God thing and All God. It is also the time that I began to write and publish books, so God did have a better plan. It was one of my hardest times in life financially and personally, but also a time I grew closer to the Lord Spiritually than ever before, so it is a time I would not trade for the world. I cashed in our 401K early with penalty to finance publishing a book and also to get out of debt. We came into this season full of debt, but came out debt free. For that I was extremely thankful, but our stable future for retirement was not a pretty picture.

There were many who lost much after the crash of 2008, many whose stocks and retirement suffered. I know my uncle had retired with a good stock portfolio before this and him and my aunt had great plans for the future and it looked good and stable. With his retirement, social security, and stock, he shouldn't have to work and they could winter in Florida with no problems. Well, he lost a lot in 2008 and both he and my aunt had to go back to work to supplement their income. He was pretty devastated at the time, but his job was mornings maintaining a golf course which when he was finished work could golf for free which is what he wanted to do anyway in retirement. They still take a couple months off a year for Florida. So things did not go perfectly as planned, but they did work out in the end.

We as seniors do have financial perks and many discounts we can use as we grow older. There are discounts meals, movies, entertainment, travel, and many other resources. There is a honor that comes with age. Many also have social security to go along with other retirement resources. There is reverse mortgage that have helped many to access funds from the homes they have worked and paid for. There are many other areas that we can save money on. It is definitely less expensive to survive when not raising a family even though I try to help my kids and grand-children any way we can.

You know, I started getting concerned with finances when I started seeing posts on Facebook from class mates retiring in Florida, taking many trips, buying new cars and living the life that the world deemed successful.

That is where we get into our most trouble when we start looking around and comparing with others. Comparing ourselves to others means we are looking the wrong way. We are looking outward when we should always be looking upward. There are always going to be those who have more and those who have less. The Bible says; "God supplies all our needs according to his riches in Glory through Christ Jesus."(Philippians 4:19) All of us have needs and my needs, wants, and desires have always been met by God. God supplies because everything is his. "Indeed heaven and the highest heavens belong to the Lord your God, also the earth and all that is in it." (Deuteronomy 10:14) For by him all things were created, that are in the heaven, and that are in the earth; all things were created by him and for him." (Colossians 1:16) The houses, land, wealth, goods, stores, automobiles, and anything else you can think of belongs to God.

Truth is, if you live in the United States of America have a car and house, sleep in a bed, and have enough food, you are one of the top twenty five percent wealthiest people in the world. We have taken all the Lord have given us for granted. That is what it means to be in the world when we are consumed by our worldly lusts of fame and fortune instead of by what kind of person and what good we can do for others. We in the United States have become UN-thankful, UN-holy, and selfish. There is such an entitlement spirit in this nation, people believing they deserve whatever they desire without even lifting a finger to earn it. We are a Blessed nation and a Blessed people. We are stewards of all we have been given. I believe I will be able to stand before God at the throne and say I have used what I have been given for the benefit of my family but also the benefit of others. There are many who have much more than I do and I hope they can say they can stand before the throne with a pure heart. I do not want to stand before God and him say look at all that was given and you wicked and lazy servant have kept all for your own. I want him to say; "Thou good and faithful servant, you have been faithful in much, enter into the Joy of the Lord." (Matthew 25:14-30) The Lord has been more than faithful to me and the least I can do for him is to be faithful to him for his salvation, his grace, his blessings, and to use it to advance his kingdom and his plan.

Well that was my "religious rant" for the book. It is not just religious, but has a lot of merit and truth to it. I do not want to get into the place and position of selfishness or being UN-thankful. Truth is many years ago, God couldn't have given me wealth because of where I was, I probably would have spent it on myself. God has poured into me grace and I know what ever else he pours into me I will be a faithful steward with it. When he pours grace and love into you, you have the perfect giving heart. My life verse is "Trust in the Lord with all your heart and lean not on your own understanding; in all your ways acknowledge him and he will direct your paths." (Proverbs 3:5-6) The Lord placed this in my mind, my heart, and my spirit even before I knew this was in the Bible. That is how I knew it was my life verse. Yours will probably be different but you will know it when the Spirit of God gives it to you. The Lord has based my life, and directed me to live my life according to this verse. He wants me to Trust first and foremost, to receive of his wisdom, to acknowledge him where ever I am, whatever I am doing, and to whom I meet.

We said at the beginning of this book that emotional strength was a combination of mind, will, and emotions. This chapter to this point was more about mind, thoughts, and concerns where finances seemed to be the biggest subject matter, now we will move into the area of our heart. The heart and the state of our own heart is one of the most important things in life. We get consumed with the mind and thoughts but the heart is where we give, have compassion, and love. "As a man thinks in his heart, so is he." (Proverbs 23:7) Our true self and our true character all come from our heart. Our mind can play tricks on us sometimes and deceive us, but our heart is truth. The Word of God discerns the thoughts and intentions of the heart. (Hebrews 4:12) See, our heart has thoughts also. Our hearts reveal our meditations and our methods. We may be able to fool some with our words and actions, but our heart reveals who we really are, to God and to others, and even to ourselves. "Out of the abundance of our heart, our mouth speaks." (Matthew 12:34) Listen to your self or others closely, after a period of time just through their speaking you will know what is in their heart and what kind of person they are.

The thing that consumes my thoughts and more of our heart is our family. That was probably true in other life seasons, but I think more in this one. Do your realize that in God's eyes that family, just like our bodies described in the previous chapter is a temple to our Lord. Our four children and seven grandchildren are all out of our home and on their own. We are extremely blessed that three of our children and our grandchildren are all within fifty miles. Psalm 127 reads; "Children are a heritage of the Lord, as arrows in the hand of a mighty man, so are the children of our youth, happy is the man who has his quiver full of them." Our quiver and our heritage and our legacy passed down is full and we are extremely blessed and joyful. There is nothing more important in life than a happy marriage and a large family. If you have that in life with your health you have everything.

As close as everyone is, sometimes we don't see each other as much as my wife or I would like. All of us are guilty of getting consumed with work and other responsibilities. My wife's heart is with the children and grandchildren twenty four seven. That is probably true with most women and mothers. I can remember spending a weekend away with just my wife, sipping wine and setting in a hot tub and my wife saying;

"Wouldn't be great if the kids were with us!" As a man and husband, my answer would be, NO, LOL. I do enjoy my time with the kids and grand-kids, but at that particular moment, my wife was my focus.

Now that I have opened this box of special time with my wife, I want to take a moment to write about love, intimacy, and sex. If you are able and sexually active at this age; Awesome! God said it was good when he created the earth but said it was "Very Good" when he made man and woman. Your marriage, your love, your intimacy, and special time with your life partner at this senior season is icing on the cake. One thing is for sure you have more time to invest in each other, to pamper and spoil each other without any interruptions. If you are not sexually active, there is always intimacy. Intimacy will last forever, but our sexual encounters were kind of brief even when we were younger, lol. It touches my heart and any one-else when I see a older couple holding hands, walking together, or a man with his arm around a woman especially at our age. A lot of couples at our age have a lot of history and a lot of love they have experienced and given. God said that the two (man and woman) would be one flesh when brought together in the covenant of marriage, Many who have had this long history are definitely one at this point. Some so much that when one of the partners passed, the other followed closely. Sex is a gift from God but intimacy is also if not more so. Sex is more of the physical where intimacy is more of the mind, heart, and spirit. When we have this kind of closeness with another, we know each other like no one else can. Intimacy with God is the same way, he longs to know you like no one else can and you to also know him.

The R-Rated portion being done (LOL), we can get back to family again. Our kids use the grandparents as baby sitters many times. That is just great with my wife and she loves nothing more. Although I love being with the grand-kids, my true definition of family time is with kids and grand-kids; all gathered together around the table, for picnics and cookouts, for parties and trips. That is Family Time to me and there is nothing greater. My dream and desire for all of us is take a trip together to Florida, to rent a big house we can all stay in, to spend time on the beach, to go to Disney and to just do nothing than to celebrate us as a family. See, that is where strong emotions and finances really do come together. I don't have the finances to be able to do this right now, but I am believing for it. God gives us the desires of our heart,and he knows this is our heart's desire.

Not to get caught up on finances again, but being on a budget we get creative on our times together. We make do and plan as many do on what they have. We live in Northern Michigan so there is much to do especially in the summertime. Swimming and camping are big things with our family. Cook outs and playing golf are also great during this time. We sled or snowmobile or ski in the winter sometimes depending on the temperatures. When you get below zero, it is hard for me and my wife at this age to really tolerate it. Another dream and desire for my wife and I is to be snowbirds; going to Florida January through March. Purchasing a camper will accomplish two things; being able to get away in the winter, but also having a camper to spend time with family camping. It may only be a dream right now, but I am believing it to be a reality someday. Watching the kids playing various sports and other school activities are very enjoyable for me. We all enjoy sports, but even I prefer and get more excited watching the kids than even professional sports.

I do not want anyone to assume that our family is perfect because no ones is, but that is what makes a family; imperfect people who stick it out through good times and bad. We as a family have had our ups and downs, our highs and lows, and even a couple of divorces that have shaken us to the core, but we are resilient. We find a way to make things work even in the troubled times. We know that even the hard times will pass. We know all things will work for good for those who love God and are called according to his purpose. God brought us all together for good and for a purpose. I would say that the divorces were probably the hardest times our family had gone through. That has sent our minds spinning, our emotions reeling, and our life seemingly out of control. Since we are a family full of sons and boys, we lose daughter in laws. It is hard to have a relationship for many years and to watch that get severed. We have always tried to adopt into our heart any our sons have joined together with. We have gained others and even gained additional children that we adopt in our heart, but it is a huge change. In many cases, our grandchildren we used to see all the time, we are now seeing every other week. We have to change our schedules and adopt to different schedules. We alter our plans and change our plans accordingly even based on the weeks that we see them. I am sure there are many who are reading this can relate. I am sure that your family is also filled with its ups and downs.

Grand-kids are the extension of family during our senior years that enlarges our family and enhances our family. With our kids, we may have gotten preoccupied with work and provision sometimes, but with our grandchildren we are preoccupied with who they are and what they are becoming. It is not that we did not do that with our kids, but we have more time to invest in the grand-kids. It is great that in your senior season you have more time to spend with family than you did working and forty to fifty hour week. People joke that with grand-kids you can enjoy them for a time then send them home to their parents. We miss them greatly and think about them often when not with them. We realize at this stage of life how fast time goes, how quick kids really do grow up and that even our grand children will grow up and have kids themselves. Time is in no one's hands, time moves forward constantly and continuously.

A day seems to take forever, but a lifetime goes in a moment. I can remember like it yesterday my own kids being ten, now we have grand-children ten and a couple even twenty or older who are married.

I know as I have gotten older, I also have gotten more mellow and more patient. With my kids, I was consumed on them growing up and being responsible adults, with my grand-kids I think more about and am more sensitive in what encourages them and what hurts their hearts. With my kids, I would be on them to clean their rooms and messes, but with grand-children even fingerprints on the windows are messages from Heaven. These are regrets I had when I was younger, but also things I have learned as I got older. I try to place these things in the hearts of my kids because I want them to realize how fast things go, and how quickly their kids are growing. I question and wonder if they actually hear and grasp what I am trying to say or are they just like me when I was their age. The song "Cat's in the cradle" recorded back in 1977 when I had just graduated high school was powerful and something I should have listened closer to then, but it describes many of us now.

The lyrics basically say no time now, but we will get together sometime, we will have a great time then. This goes on through many stages of life, they never get together, and it closes with "My boy was just like me!" This song talks about family, life, time, heritage, and legacy. If you are reading this as a middle age person, know that this time is precious with all members of your family also.

I said it before and will say it again, time is precious with family. You don't know how long you will have with each other. That is another thing I try to convey to my kids, that at our age we may not be around much longer. I do not confess death or proclaim it, but it happens to us all. My kids are 30-40 years old, and at thirty is when I lost my parents. I had never experienced death until that time, but from January till August of 1990 I lost my grandmother, my mother, and my father. My mother did not actually pass until Mother's Day of 1992, but she had surgical complications in 1990 that made her basically a vegetable. It was quick and it was unexpected and it was devastating. My own kids may go through this themselves and it is the hardest parts of life.

I am thankful for the time I had with my parents because there are so many who lose their parents or other close family members even at younger ages. One of my greatest losses was my brother in 2009. It was 19 years from my parents to my brother but seemed so quick. He was fifty but we went through many things together and was very close. Again,I am thankful I had him that long but I think about him often and it was probably the worse loss of my life. I do not wish this on anyone even though this happens to all of us and it happens daily to many. Although we try not to think about death, at our age it always seems to be knocking and could be around any corner. I do not fear death for myself for I know and am confident what is on the other side. But, I know it well be a hard and difficult time for my kids and other members of our family. I do not wish this on anyone but unfortunately, it is a part of life.

I am thankful for family and it is the greatest gift the Lord has given to any of us. I pray for all of you to treasure your family, wife, husband, kids, and grand-kids for they are all precious. If there are any who are having family disagreements or squabbles and have not seen each other for some time, forgive and repair and restore your relationship as quick as you can. You will wish you did if the opportunity is gone and you will be forever glad if you can look back and say you did all you could do. Your relationship with all your family is the most important relationship you can have on this earth other than your relationship with God. I want to be united with my family always in the earth, but even more want all of us to be together again in Heaven.

Chapter Four
Spiritual Strength
Legacy / Grace
"Train up a child in the way they should go"

Spiritual Strength to me is first and foremost the most important strength we can have at this stage of life. It is and has been my greatest strength in every stage of my life. It has brought me through many trials. I do not know how I would have went through some things without the benefit of the Lord walking with me and carrying me through things. I do not know how people who haven't come to the light of his salvation or refuse his offer of gift and grace do it day to day. Many think that those with religion and those who have a relationship with God the Father show signs of weakness and cannot make it on their own anyway. Being humble is not being weak, but being strong in a way you actually admit that there are times you can give help but there are also times we need help. Anyone who thinks they do not need help and encouragement at times are very prideful and not honest with themselves.

The sub-title to this book is aging with Grace. I wrote this and said this for my entire life has, was, and is being directed and corrected by Grace. Grace is defined as receiving something we have never deserved. I had an elder always keep saying years ago; "Thank God for Grace, I am amazed by His Grace." I was younger then and had some understanding for what he was saying but

I have greater understanding now and even more amazed as he was then. Many confuse Grace and Mercy at times. Mercy is not receiving a punishment, sentence, or judgment we do deserve. By Mercy we have been pardoned and set free even being guilty for so many things. On top of receiving Mercy from the Lord, the Lord has been exceptionally good to me all these years, bestowed on me Grace and Gifts and Love despite myself and my failings. Maybe that is why we are so amazed by his Grace, we keep getting blessed when our natural mind says we should be judged. I expound on Grace in another of my books. This was written way back when I heard that elder make his proclamation, and I desired more understanding.

The Book of Proverbs tells us that wisdom is the principal thing, so with all our getting to get wisdom. We talked previously that with our years we get knowledge, understanding, and wisdom, but the truth is the Bible also says that we only get wisdom by and through God. Wisdom is attained through God, age has nothing to do with it. "If any of you lack wisdom, let him ask of God, that gives to all men generously." (James 1:5) To get wisdom all we have to do is ask God. I cannot tell you all the times that God has showed me how to have a happier marriage, how to mend relationships, how to fix a problem at work, to even how to fix issues with a furnace. The list would be endless of all the wisdom I received from the Lord over the years.

He gave it to me whenever I asked and he will also give it to you.

I was brought up Catholic where I felt we had religion but really did not know God. I didn't feel I could get close to the priest who we sat on pedestals much less the God we preached. I wasn't even sure there was a God until I met him personally in 1998, the year I was born again. I was 41 years old at the time. I was sure grateful that with all the mistakes and sins I had committed to that point were not held against me, and there were many. I was a selfish person and as I looked back on it, pretty evil to the core and deserving of hell fire. I asked the Lord into my heart, met the Holy Spirit of God and knew without a shadow of a doubt that there was a God. Talk about your heart leaping and dancing, I was in seventh Heaven. I had searched years for purpose and to fill that emptiness and questions I had in my heart and mind and it was answered. In fact, the whole family was born again and baptized together in April of 1998. Salvation was instant, but sanctification is a process; a process of getting to know God more, becoming closer to Him and becoming like Him. Learning what is important to God through His Word, the Bible, and through prayer, meditation, and reflection. God speaks in many ways and he will speak to you and through many ways. If we take the time and make the time for God, he will draw close to you and make his ways known. After being born again, I couldn't get enough of the Word, but I had a lot of religion to unlearn.

There may be many who do not understand what it means to be born again. A lot of it is spiritual so a little difficult to explain until you experience it personally. I became born again when I repented of my sins and accepted Jesus into my heart. That was a spiritual cleansing of my past but also a renewal in my heart and spirit. The other thing that happened shortly after this confession was that I was baptized. Baptism is basically an outward confession of an inward regeneration. When baptized we are submersed in water to signify the death of Christ, but also the death of our old man. When we are raise from the water we signify the resurrection of Christ but also our resurrection to a new man. It is just like you are born again into new life. That is great news especially in our senior season, our old man dies, and the new man lives.

The thing that was even greater than being born again was being born again as a family. As a family we were learning and growing in the Lord. The greatest thing I am proud of as a father is that I passed faith to my children. I passed on devotion to God through example. They learned that although I had faults and failures, I still had and have faith. One thing one of my sons says he respects and remembers about me is that I had devotions and bible in hand every mourning. I tried to pass faith on to my children, but realized as the years go by, that they still had to have their own faith. Even though some of my children do not attend Church weekly, they still have the root and foundation of faith.

The Bible says and I believe and stand on it; "Train up a child in the way they should go and they will not depart from it." (Proverbs 22:6) See, another instruction from the Book of Proverbs, the Book of Wisdom. If you plant this seed, the root and foundation will grow. We may help our children in the act of faith, but it is there responsibility to make faith grow. Actually what is better news evidenced by our scripture above our children do not depart because not only have they been trained, but our Lord will continue to pursue them. Their faith becomes God's responsibility who is always faithful.

The other thing that is awesome through this that it not only gets passed to your children but also your children's children, your grand-children. That is my greatest pride and my greatest legacy. Everyone wants to be known for something. We crave a sense of significance. Something in us tells us our lives were not in vain and that we made a difference on this earth. We are to leave our children and grandchildren an inheritance, but more importantly we leave them a legacy. "A good man leaves an inheritance to his children's children." (Proverbs 13:22) We as followers of the Lord when talking on finances should be able to leave not only enough for our children, but also our grandchildren. When I leave to my children our house, bank accounts and personal items I am leaving an inheritance. As important and valuable as that is, leaving a legacy is more important. When I model a devotion to God, an example of faith, a respect and devotion to their mother, a great work ethic and honesty, we are leaving a legacy which has much more value. An inheritance may last through their life here on earth, but a legacy will last through eternity. We think we need to make a great contribution to make a difference here on earth, but the truth is every relationship, every gift, every encouragement, and every service we do makes a difference and not only affects the one but the thousands that person touches. We do not do things for reward but your reward in Heaven will be greater than you could have imagined through the daily things.

I know there are many who are reading this may argue and say, "I have known many who have had great inheritance, and family, and wealth without religion and without having a relationship with the Lord. I would say you probably have and there are some on the earth without a relationship who have by worldly terms been good people and have been successes. There has even been those who have accumulated much through lies, deceit, drugs or pornography. Many questions that I cannot even answer. That is just one of the great things about God, he gives all free will to choose him or not. It rains on the just and the unjust. God is not involved in all the evil that goes on, nor is he blind to it, but there are many that will answer to him for their life and the way they lived their life in due time and season.

I know some believe that they will just die, be buried, and that is the end of life. Because of my relationship with God, I know that to not be true no matter how much those want to deny or reject him. At the end there is a judgment for all people and the way they lived their lives. I assure you there is a God in Heaven who has all things under his control. There is a Heaven and there is a Hell. There is a story in the Bible about a rich man and a poor man. (Luke 16) The rich man had everything he wanted on the earth, and the poor man ate from the crumbs of the rich man's table. That wasn't just or right but it still happened. Upon their death, the rich man went to hell and the poor man to Heaven. The rich man seeing Heaven from Hell asked Abraham to send the poor man with a drop of cool water because he was tormented in Hell. (Weird those in Hell can see those in Heaven, but not the opposite, just part of the torment). The rich man's next request was that his brothers and family to be warned of the place called Hell. The rich man did not want his family to end up in that place. He may have had a great inheritance but his legacy did not mean much at this time. His primary concern was that his family would be in Heaven. That is my concern with all my family and my concern for writing this book and for all those who may read this book. There is a place reserved in Heaven for all who have made Jesus their Lord and Savior. There is also a place reserved in Hell for those who haven't.

I do not know or have all the answers of why certain things are on this earth or why some prosper and others do not. All I know there is good and evil, right and wrong, righteousness and UN-righteousness. All I know is that everyone has sinned and fallen short of the glory of God. The Bible says that there is no one good, no not one. (Psalm 14:3 / Romans 3:12) If we are in the earth, we have all sinned and anyone who has sinned deserves judgment. We can try to fool others around us that we are good people and have not sinned. You are trying to tell others and yourselves that you have not lied, stolen, or killed. The Bible says that if you are angry with another and have not forgiven another, you have killed,and your Father in Heaven cannot forgive you. But your Father in Heaven has provided a way for forgiveness, mercy, and salvation. He sent his one and only son Jesus to die in your place for your sin. Jesus paid a debt he did not owe so you could be redeemed and be with Him forever. Jesus is the way, the truth, and the Life; no one comes to the Father without him. (John 14:6) The way has been provided and that way is Jesus. Any other way is a deception and a lie. This is the truth that I know that I know.

Spiritual Strength is my approach to life each and every day. Spiritual strength is peace and joy in the midst of trial and tribulation. Not rejoicing in difficult times, but rejoicing that there is one who is above all that, who has me in his capable hands, and who is faithful to me, my wife, and my family. We were chosen before the foundation of the earth, and so are you. God's ultimate will is that none perish but come to the knowledge of his Truth. His will is none would enter

Hell, Hell was created only for the devil and his angels, but there is spiritual principal in the earth when sin entered the earth. Hell is for those who choose to follow their worldly lusts and sin.

There is no unrighteousness in Heaven. You have to understand the pure holiness of our God. He cannot be in the presence of sin, even though he sees all of the sin going on in the earth. By the blood sacrifice of his son and by accepting that sacrifice we are washed and cleansed as if we have never sinned. "Without the shedding of blood, there is no remission of sin (pardon/freedom)." (Hebrews 9:22) But Jesus shed his blood on that cross for us to be cleansed and free from sin. Jesus provided a way for us to the Father and to Heaven. He gave the ultimate sacrifice and paid the penalty for our sins. He paid a debt he did not owe, our debt and our judgment.

This is the only way to eternal life. I know that many who are reading this are in their senior season, those of the age of sixty or more. I received Jesus as Savior at forty, but if your are reading this now, you have the opportunity to receive him in your sixties. I am glad that I got to know Jesus, but always wish I knew him sooner. Either way, it isn't when you receive, just that you do. If you are reading this, you have the opportunity and the door is open now. There is nothing hindering you from receiving God and all his Goodness, but You. We get prideful in our age and stuck in our ways, but do not let that keep you from the most wonderful thing on this earth; Salvation through Jesus Christ.

"A beautiful face will age and a perfect body will change, but a beautiful soul will always be a beautiful soul." (Author Unknown)